THE EVENING MEDITATION JOURNAL

THE EVENING MEDITATION JOURNAL

Relaxing Prompts for Reflection and Relaxation

Worthy Stokes

R

ROCKRIDGE
PRESS

Interior and Cover Designer: Lisa Forde
Art Producer: Hannah Dickerson
Editor: John Makowski
Author photo courtesy of David Genik Photography
ISBN: Print 978-1-64876-987-0 | eBook 978-1-64876-988-7
R0

THIS JOURNAL BELONGS TO

_____

"It is your light that lights the world."

RUMI

INTRODUCTION

Welcome to *The Evening Meditation Journal*, your gentle guide to practicing mindful gratitude, reflective inspiration, and writing as an act of restorative self-care. Perhaps you picked up this book because you're feeling stressed and anxious, or maybe you have been struggling privately in your efforts to let go of worries, gain perspective, or experience deep rest. Whether you hope to develop a completely new meditation practice or deepen a current one, this journal is designed to support your journey within. As you take time to close each day with heartfelt intention, your sleep will improve, your relationship with yourself will be nourished, and your waking life will transform.

My name is Worthy Stokes. I have been teaching meditation and coaching clients since 2018, although my personal meditation practice began 10 years prior. Having practiced everything from one-hour sits and recitations of mantras to weeks of solitary retreat in total silence, I have prepared this journal for you in a way that distills what is essential. Every practice is carefully designed to illuminate and nurture your magnificent potential at the nexus of science, soma, and soul.

The Power of Rest

An evening meditation practice directly supports wellness by helping you nurture your innermost awareness and empowering you to heal. Research shows the strength of one's immune system is closely linked to quality of sleep, so a meditation routine may dramatically improve your physical health. By leveraging your body's natural instinct to restore itself, evenings can be transformed into a time of self-care.

How to Use This Journal

The Evening Meditation Journal is designed to be used in a way that feels comfortable and relaxed. It is also a gentle invitation to establish a regular evening meditation and journaling practice. You will see the most transformation if you choose to practice daily, at the same time every evening, because research shows that meditating for five minutes a day is more than enough to make a measurable difference. That said, it is perfectly fine to practice weekly, or at random, as inspired.

EVENING MEDITATION PRACTICES

Every evening starts with a short, guided mindfulness meditation exercise to help you relax and connect to a mindful flow and state of relaxation. Each practice is gentle, easy to follow, and designed to take approximately five minutes.

JOURNAL PROMPTS FOR SELF-REFLECTION

There are three brief journal prompts that accompany each practice. By meditating *and* journaling, you are better able to integrate mindful awareness with cognitive attention and somatic intuition.

EXPRESSING GRATITUDE

By regularly expressing gratitude, you bring a sense of your innate worthiness to your life. The simple choice to consciously attune to gratitude every evening will help you build new neural networks, sculpt your consciousness, and strengthen your resilience.

I congratulate you for giving yourself the transformative gift of self-care, and I hope you find the peace, clarity, and rest you seek. May you be happy, healthy, and at ease with this life.

DAY 1

HUGGING MEDITATION FOR SELF-LOVE

Choose a comfortable position you can maintain for several moments. Inhale and exhale slowly as you wrap your arms around yourself in a gentle, loving hug. With every inhalation and every exhalation, tune in to a soothing warmth within. Hold yourself in a caring embrace for as long as you feel is natural. Connect with a sense of feeling deeply held and enjoy the quiet benefit of offering yourself kindhearted presence.

1. Describe the feeling of the hug you gave to yourself.

_____

_____

_____

_____

2. How does it feel to show yourself love?

_____

_____

_____

_____

3. Notice how you felt before and after this meditation. What differences do you sense?

_____

_____

_____

_____

THREE THINGS I AM GRATEFUL FOR TODAY:

1. _____

2. _____

3. _____

DAY 2

RADICAL ACCEPTANCE (OF WHAT YOU CANNOT CHANGE)

By practicing presence with something that cannot be changed, you cultivate a powerful ability to harness the positive effects of radical acceptance. Center yourself with several breaths. Reflect on your day and think of something you wish you had done differently; bring it to your mind's eye. With each inhalation, embrace this thing you cannot change with acceptance. With every exhalation, gently let it go. Feel yourself become lighter with each breath as you release today with gentle ease.

1. How can accepting what you cannot change help you feel more relaxed?

_____

_____

_____

_____

2. What do you notice when you center yourself in radical acceptance?

_____

_____

_____

_____

3. After giving yourself permission to release today, are you able to feel more at ease?

_____

_____

_____

_____

THREE THINGS I AM GRATEFUL FOR TODAY:

1. _____

2. _____

3. _____

DAY 3

VISUALIZATION FOR CALM SLEEP

By visualizing an abiding presence of inner peace, you can utilize this sacred resource anytime you wish. Prepare for calm sleep by gently turning your attention inward. Set an intention to rest in restorative awareness. Visualize a warm, easy current of light as you dip into the quiet reserves of your inner-most landscape and gently connect with an expansive, internal calm. Invite the strength of your inner peace to hold you in this clear, soft illumination.

1. When you envision calm sleep, what comes to mind?

_____

_____

_____

_____

2. Even when you experience stress, are you able to sense your inner-most strength?

_____

_____

_____

_____

3. What can you do, in this very moment, to bring a calm sense of presence to your evening?

_____

_____

_____

_____

THREE THINGS I AM GRATEFUL FOR TODAY:

1. _____

2. _____

3. _____

DAY 4

THE SWEET SPACE OF GRATITUDE

Breathing through your nose with your mouth closed, reflect on your day; think of one simple thing you feel grateful for. It can be as simple as a warm cup of tea or an open, sunny sky. With every inhale and exhale, quietly think to yourself, *thank you, thank you, thank you*, until you feel complete. Give yourself permission to connect, over and over again, with the sweet space of gratitude.

1. What does gratitude mean to you?

_____

_____

_____

_____

2. Notice how a meditation on gratitude feels in your body. What changed?

_____

_____

_____

_____

3. How can you incorporate more gratitude into your life?

_____

_____

_____

_____

THREE THINGS I AM GRATEFUL FOR TODAY:

1. _____

2. _____

3. _____

DAY 5

EVENING BODY SCAN FOR RELAXATION

1. Lie down and close your eyes.

2. Begin by breathing naturally, then start scanning your body for sensations.

3. As you inhale, deliberately tense your muscles.

4. As you exhale, gently release this tension.

5. As you continue to breathe mindfully for several moments, repeat this process and observe the parts of your body that begin to relax.

6. Continue to breathe mindfully for several moments.

1. Where does your body often hold tension?

_____

_____

_____

_____

2. How does mindful breathing change that tension?

_____

_____

_____

_____

3. As you scan your internal environment, reflect on how kind you are to yourself.

_____

_____

_____

_____

THREE THINGS I AM GRATEFUL FOR TODAY:

1. _____

2. _____

3. _____

DAY 6

LET YOUR GRIEF REST

Settle into a comfortable position of ease and reflect on any sensations you may have of sadness, grief, or loss. Breathing naturally, gently inhale and exhale. Imagine a warm and gentle space emerging in the center of your mind's eye. As this space gradually expands, tune in to the parts of your body where the feeling of grief resides. Mentally invite any of these sensations to be fully present. Let your grief soften and rest in this warm, spacious awareness.

1. What is a gentle way to offer support when you or someone you love is grieving?

_____

_____

_____

_____

2. Do you give yourself ample time and space to grieve? To rest?

_____

_____

_____

_____

3. In what way can you better support yourself when feelings of sadness arise?

_____

_____

_____

_____

THREE THINGS I AM GRATEFUL FOR TODAY:

1. _____

2. _____

3. _____

DAY 7

YOUR INNER RIVER OF HEALING QUIETUDE

Relax your fingers, loosen your jaw, and settle into the good medicine of your very own presence. As you soften your gaze or close your eyes, connect with the silence within. Imagine a tender river of quietude moving through your bloodstream, gently massaging your cells, bones, and breath. As you sense this inner river of healing moving through you, let it carry you into sleep and your dreaming landscape with ease and grace.

1. How does it feel to know there is a river of self-healing energy you can access anytime?

_____

_____

_____

_____

2. What do you notice when you stop to acknowledge the healing potential of your own presence?

_____

_____

_____

_____

3. Describe what comes to mind when you think of the word "grace."

_____

_____

_____

_____

THREE THINGS I AM GRATEFUL FOR TODAY:

1. _____

2. _____

3. _____

DAY 8

HUNGER IS A MESSENGER

Take a moment to reflect on what you need to feel nourished, safe, and at ease this evening. Recall the care you took today with sensations of hunger. Is your hunger spiritual? Is it physical? Make contact with your innermost holy sense of longing, and with every exhale, release self-judgment. With every inhale, invite your body to feel weightless, as if you are grounded in space. Hunger is a sacred messenger; let it breathe.

1. Describe your relationship to longing. Do you give yourself permission to experience desire?

_____

_____

_____

_____

2. If your hunger could speak, what would it say it needs?

_____

_____

_____

_____

3. How do you feel about taking up space in ways that are healthy, joyful, and inspiring?

_____

_____

_____

_____

THREE THINGS I AM GRATEFUL FOR TODAY:

1. _____

2. _____

3. _____

DAY 9

LOVING-KINDNESS MEDITATION
FOR HEALTH AND WELLNESS

While sitting quietly or lying down, repeat the following for several moments to expand loving-kindness: *May I be happy. May I be healthy. May I be at ease with this life.* Next, think of a loved one suffering or in pain. While holding this person in your thoughts, repeat the practice: *May you be happy. May you be healthy. May you be at ease with this life.* Invite this practice of prayerful generosity to soothe you.

1. Reflect on the way this meditation feels; describe the sensations you notice.

_____

_____

_____

_____

2. When offering this prayer to yourself, does anything in you change?

_____

_____

_____

_____

3. When offering this prayer to another person, does anything
   in you change?

_____

_____

_____

_____

THREE THINGS I AM GRATEFUL FOR TODAY:

1. _____

2. _____

3. _____

DAY 10

GENTLE SONIC HEALING MEDITATION

Organize a playlist of songs you feel are gentle, comforting, and soft, then choose its title. For example: *Evening Meditation Music for Healing*. Find a comfortable place to rest, start your playlist, and practice the contemplative art of deep listening. Imagine you are being wrapped in a healing sonic hug as you rest in comforting waves of sound. Notice how an acoustic landscape can hold you with gentle ease and amplify resonance.

1. Is sound an effective way for you to self-soothe?

_____

_____

_____

_____

2. Describe your acoustic landscape and why you chose these songs.

_____

_____

_____

_____

3. How does music impact your sense of well-being?

_____

_____

_____

_____

THREE THINGS I AM GRATEFUL FOR TODAY:

1. _____

2. _____

3. _____

DAY 11

AH OM HUNG RAM DZA: TIBETAN MANTRA PRACTICE

1. Visualize white light and connect with vast inner space as you chant a long *AH*.

2. Visualize the color yellow and connect with compassionate communication as you chant *OM*.

3. Visualize the color green and feel the warmth of healing as you chant *HUNG*.

4. Visualize the color red and connect with your personal power as you chant *RAM*.

5. Complete the practice by visualizing the color blue and connecting with your ability to transform your deepest wisdom into action as you chant *DZA*.

1. Which syllable did you connect with most and why?

_____

_____

_____

_____

2. What would you like to bring more healing energy to in the coming days?

_____

_____

_____

_____

3. Do you feel more open and spacious after this practice?

_____

_____

_____

_____

THREE THINGS I AM GRATEFUL FOR TODAY:

1. _____

2. _____

3. _____

DAY 12

OPEN AWARENESS FOR RELAXATION

Settle in for a gentle practice of nondirective attention known as "open awareness." As you rest your body and mind, abide with what is. Allow thoughts, feelings, or physical sensations from the day to arise and remain without judgment. This is a gentle practice of awakening to the subtle qualities of attention, where there is nothing to do or accomplish; in staying open and aware, you become more present and more relaxed, from one moment of your evening to the next.

1. Take time to reflect on the practice of letting your mind be busy, active, and inspired.

_____

_____

_____

_____

2. Did you enjoy this practice, or do you prefer a more focused type of meditation?

_____

_____

_____

_____

3. How can awakening to subtle qualities of attention help prepare you for a restful evening?

_____

_____

_____

_____

THREE THINGS I AM GRATEFUL FOR TODAY:

1. _____

2. _____

3. _____

DAY 13

HEARTMIND® VISUALIZATION

While placing your hands over your heart and turning your attention inward, offer a quiet prayer of gratitude for your ability to think, feel, and transform, from your soul to every cell in your body. With your eyes softly closed, visualize your mind illuminated with light. Next, visualize your heart illuminated with light, so both your mind and your heart radiate soft luminosity together. Last, visualize your breath illuminated with light. Ease into your felt sense of HeartMind® connection.

1. What sensations did you notice after connecting your heart, mind, and breath?

_____

_____

_____

_____

2. How does visualization help you integrate a felt sense of awareness in your body?

_____

_____

_____

_____

3. Describe your experience with the healing light in this meditation.

_____

_____

_____

_____

THREE THINGS I AM GRATEFUL FOR TODAY:

1. _____

2. _____

3. _____

DAY 14

INNER SMILE FOR DISSOLVING TENSION

Begin by closing your eyes and relaxing your whole body. Breathing naturally, connect with your inner landscape and loosen the muscles of your face, hands, and toes. As you soften naturally, reflect on something from your day that brought or brings you joy, and smile from the inside, without moving your face *at all*. Can you feel the warmth of your inner smile? Let this inner smile dissolve any sensation of tension that remains from your day.

1. Were you able to feel the warmth of your inner smile? Describe it below.

_____

_____

_____

_____

2. If you practice this inner-smile meditation when you feel upset, what might happen?

_____

_____

_____

_____

3. Could you keep a straight face during this practice, or did you start smiling?

_____

_____

_____

_____

THREE THINGS I AM GRATEFUL FOR TODAY:

1. _____

2. _____

3. _____

DAY 15

HOW TO BEFRIEND YOUR ANXIETY

By befriending anxiety, you can learn to self-soothe when feeling overwhelmed. As anxiety arrives, treat it as a cherished lost friend. Find a comfortable position and gently shift your awareness to your breath, inhaling and exhaling with fluidity and ease. Instead of judging thoughts or feelings of anxiety from the day, let it all rest *inside* your breath. Experiment with perceiving anxiety as a lonely friend longing for comfort. Notice whether mindful breathing helps you self-soothe and settle from within.

1. What changes when you approach anxiety as a friend instead of an enemy?

_____

_____

_____

_____

2. How does mindful breathing help?

_____

_____

_____

_____

3. Describe the way your anxiety feels after befriending it.

_____

_____

_____

_____

THREE THINGS I AM GRATEFUL FOR TODAY:

1. _____

2. _____

3. _____

DAY 16

THE ART OF NOTICING PEACE

1. The art of noticing peace is a mindfulness practice you can use anytime.

2. While reflecting on your day, recall what was peaceful in someone you met, or acknowledge a peaceful element of your environment. Allow yourself to be open to the memory of this peace.

3. Take a moment to look around where you are now.

4. Notice one simple thing you find peaceful in this moment, just as it is.

5. Practice attuning to what is peaceful, and let your thinking mind rest.

1. By noticing what is peaceful, do you in turn feel more peaceful?

_____

_____

_____

_____

2. What was the most peaceful part of your day?

_____

_____

_____

_____

3. What can you see now that you might have missed if you hadn't slowed down just now?

_____

_____

_____

_____

THREE THINGS I AM GRATEFUL FOR TODAY:

1. _____

2. _____

3. _____

DAY 17

PRACTICE RAIN FOR GENTLE SLEEP

By using a framework known as RAIN, developed by Michele McDonald and popularized by psychologist and meditation teacher Tara Brach, you can prepare for gentle sleep by following these four meditation cues: *Recognize* what is happening around you, or a feeling inside you. *Accept* the experience to occur without judging it. *Investigate* the moment for what it is, with interest and care. *Nurture* your inner landscape and practice self-compassion.

As you prepare for sleep, bring this consciousness of awakened self-love into your dreaming space, and rest.

1. Describe what sensations you noticed and how it felt to allow a particular feeling to arise.

_____

_____

_____

_____

2. What did you learn or discover when you investigated the present moment?

_____

_____

_____

_____

3. What comes to mind when you choose to nurture yourself with self-compassion?

_____

_____

_____

_____

THREE THINGS I AM GRATEFUL FOR TODAY:

1. _____

2. _____

3. _____

DAY 18

HUG EMOTIONAL PAIN WITH KINDHEARTEDNESS

When we push away our pain, we sometimes make the pain more painful. Let's practice hugging our pain instead. Inhale and exhale slowly as you wrap your arms around yourself in a gentle embrace. Invite any emotional pain to join you in this hug and envelop it with tender awareness. As you inhale and exhale, visualize this powerful hug embracing your pain with soothing warmth. Allow your pain to feel deeply held in kindheartedness.

1. Reflect on this meditation practice. What changed?

_____

_____

_____

_____

2. Describe the sensations you noticed when hugging your own pain with warmth.

_____

_____

_____

_____

3. As you continue to hold your pain in kindheartedness, what comes to mind?

_____

_____

_____

_____

THREE THINGS I AM GRATEFUL FOR TODAY:

1. _____

2. _____

3. _____

DAY 19

YOUR BODY IS A SANCTUARY
OF SELF-COMPASSION

Invite a sense of well-being into this moment; connect with quiet, inner wisdom. Place your hands over your heart, and with your eyes softly closed, visualize your heart space illuminated with light. Invite the vast, luminous presence of compassion to radiate from the center of your heart, then invite this luminosity to fill your entire physical body. As you breathe, notice as your whole body begins to glimmer; you are a breathing sanctuary of self-compassion.

1. What does it feel like to explore your body as a sanctuary of self-compassion?

_____

_____

_____

_____

2. When you take time to connect with inner wisdom, what happens?

_____

_____

_____

_____

3. Describe the relationship between your breath and your heart.

_____

_____

_____

_____

THREE THINGS I AM GRATEFUL FOR TODAY:

1. _____

2. _____

3. _____

DAY 20

MEDITATION FOR EXPANDING INTERNAL STRENGTH

Gently close your eyes and bring awareness to the breath. Resting with your mouth closed, inhale and exhale quietly through your nose. Notice parts of your body that feel strong, clear, and wise. Bring awareness to that strength, and invite it to expand slowly, beyond your body, into the universe, where your strongest self can take up as much space as you can imagine. With every breath, feel your innate strength expanding into infinite presence.

1. Describe one of your strengths that you appreciate.

_____

_____

_____

_____

2. How does focusing on your strength orient your mind?

_____

_____

_____

_____

3. How can you take up more space in ways that feel safe, clear, and wise?

_____

_____

_____

_____

THREE THINGS I AM GRATEFUL FOR TODAY:

1. _____

2. _____

3. _____

DAY 21

SELF-SOOTHE WITH GRATITUDE

Bring your attention to your breath. As you inhale and exhale, invite your breath to be fluid while reflecting on something you appreciate about yourself. While holding gratitude for yourself in your mind's eye, invite your felt sense of gratitude to float in a space of gentle awareness that rests in the center of your forehead. With every inhale, grant yourself permission to feel touched by your presence; give this gratitude permission to breathe.

1. What does gratitude feel like to you?

_____

_____

_____

_____

2. When offering gratitude to yourself, what do you notice?

_____

_____

_____

_____

3. How can you remind yourself to appreciate yourself more often?

_____

_____

_____

_____

THREE THINGS I AM GRATEFUL FOR TODAY:

1. _____

2. _____

3. _____

DAY 22

LEAN INTO WHAT IS GOOD

The creative energy we use for problem solving, or conflict, can be regenerated (or gently redirected) by practicing the fine art of leaning into what is good *right now*. In a comfortable position with your hands resting wherever you wish, begin to breathe naturally and effortlessly through your nose, and think of something that is good right now, in this very moment. With every inhale and exhale, release the stress of today; lean into what is good.

1. Reflect on how it felt to lean into what is good in this moment.

_____

_____

_____

_____

2. When you released the past and attuned to your present experience, what did you discover?

_____

_____

_____

_____

3. How can you continue this practice going forward?

_____

_____

_____

_____

THREE THINGS I AM GRATEFUL FOR TODAY:

1. _____

2. _____

3. _____

CELEBRATE POTENTIAL

It is natural to strive for perfection, yet part of the elegant potential of our nature as human beings is discovered in the ongoing path of revision. In other words, with every experience, mistake, or failure, we learn more about what we need to grow and transform. Take time to center yourself in the remarkable potential of your changeable nature. Give yourself permission to celebrate your human potential this evening, and as often as you can. Perfection is irrelevant.

1. What did you learn today from a mistake that you or someone else made?

_____

_____

_____

_____

2. If you trade perfectionism for the idea of making revisions, how does that feel different?

_____

_____

_____

_____

3. Describe an aspect of untapped potential that you hope to expand
in the future.

_____

_____

_____

_____

THREE THINGS I AM GRATEFUL FOR TODAY:

1. _____

2. _____

3. _____

DAY 24

INHALE PEACE AND EXHALE STRESS

Soften your gaze or close your eyes, then bring awareness to your breath and settle into an easy, natural rhythm. Resting with your mouth closed, inhale and exhale effortlessly (through your nose). As you tune in to your breath, connect with a sense of peace. Now, bring your awareness back to the present moment. Notice this clear, gentle presence. Allow the stress of the day to exit through your breath and dissolve.

1. Reflect on what peace feels like to you in your body.

_____

_____

_____

_____

2. When you exhale stress and inhale peace, what happens to your breath?

_____

_____

_____

_____

3. How does it feel to give yourself permission to rest?

_____

_____

_____

_____

THREE THINGS I AM GRATEFUL FOR TODAY:

1. _____

2. _____

3. _____

DAY 25

MEDITATION FOR SPONTANEOUS HEALING

Imagine a soft white light enveloping your entire being. As you rest in the warmth of this gentle healing energy, notice what its luminosity feels like. Does it have a texture, a weight, or a temperature? What sensations are you aware of? Remain cocooned in this space as long as you wish. Invite the very cells of your being to open to the possibility of spontaneous healing.

1. What shifts when you open yourself to the possibility of spontaneous healing?

_____

_____

_____

_____

2. What images come to mind after completing this meditation?

_____

_____

_____

_____

3. Are you aware of any changes in physical or emotional sensations?

_____

_____

_____

_____

THREE THINGS I AM GRATEFUL FOR TODAY:

1. _____

2. _____

3. _____

DAY 26

TETHER YOURSELF TO YOUR SOUL WITH LIGHT

Imagine a space behind your mind's eye. As this space expands, fill it with a soft, warm luminosity. Rest in this awareness and notice any colors or images that may arise. Envision this healing energy illuminating you from within, so you are both emanating and absorbing the presence of your nonphysical self. Imagine a thread of light connecting your soul to your body. Notice what sensations or emotions arise as you tether yourself to your soul.

1. What colors or images emerged in your mind's eye?

_____

_____

_____

_____

2. Describe how it feels to reconnect with your soul.

_____

_____

_____

_____

3. How can you maintain this connection with your soul?

_____

_____

_____

_____

THREE THINGS I AM GRATEFUL FOR TODAY:

1. _____

2. _____

3. _____

PEACE WITH DEATH, JOY WITH LIFE

1. Invite a sense of peace into your evening.

2. Resting your palms wherever you wish, begin to inhale and exhale gently. Notice your deep, abiding strength as you center yourself in your breath.

3. Repeat the following quietly for several moments: *May I be at peace with this life. May I be at ease with impermanence. May I face death with courage. May I feel joy for this life*.

4. Notice your deep, abiding strength. Center yourself in your breath.

5. Bring your awareness back to this peace whenever you wish.

1. Describe what courage feels like to you.

_____

_____

_____

_____

2. How can impermanence inspire you to be more joyful in the moment?

_____

_____

_____

_____

3. What fear about death do you need to honor and hold with tenderness?

_____

_____

_____

_____

THREE THINGS I AM GRATEFUL FOR TODAY:

1. _____

2. _____

3. _____

DAY 28

COHERENT BREATHING FOR CHRONIC PAIN

1. This practice can be done while sitting or lying down. Choose a comfortable position and soften any tension, allowing any negative thoughts to dissolve. Connect with your breath.

2. With your mouth closed, gently inhale through your nose as you count to six.

3. With your mouth closed, gently exhale through your nose as you count to six.

4. Repeat this breathing technique for five minutes.

1. What thoughts, if any, arose during this practice?

_____

_____

_____

_____

2. Do you notice a physical difference in your body after this practice?

_____

_____

_____

_____

3. How does your relationship with pain change when you rest in the power of your breath?

_____

_____

_____

_____

THREE THINGS I AM GRATEFUL FOR TODAY:

1. _____

2. _____

3. _____

DAY 29

VISUALIZATION FOR A CONFIDENT SELF-IMAGE

Visualize a space behind your mind's eye and imagine the most confident version of yourself at the top of a spiral staircase with 27 steps. Begin walking up. Give yourself permission to transform with ease, and as you climb, count backward with every step up, from 27 to 1. When you reach the final step at number 1, notice newfound confidence emerge, then gently bring your awareness back to the present moment.

1. Describe your most confident self.

_____

_____

_____

_____

2. What did you notice when you met a version of yourself that you can envision?

_____

_____

_____

_____

3. How can you embody confidence in small, manageable ways in order to build a positive self-image?

_____

_____

_____

_____

THREE THINGS I AM GRATEFUL FOR TODAY:

1. _____

2. _____

3. _____

DAY 30

ATTUNE YOURSELF TO GRACE

In a seated position, rest your hands wherever you wish. Breathing through your nose with your mouth closed, tune in to your inner space and invite a felt sense of grace to rest in the center of your mind's eye. Reflect on moments of stress during your day and notice specific moments in which you were supported without realizing it, an act of generosity you received from another person, or a sensation of wonder. Embody feelings of gratitude as you attune yourself to grace.

1. Describe a moment of your day in which you now realize you were being supported.

_____

_____

_____

_____

2. Do you take time to tune in to the subtle ways you're supported from one day to the next?

_____

_____

_____

_____

3. How can an experience of wonder be a source of support?

_____

_____

_____

_____

THREE THINGS I AM GRATEFUL FOR TODAY:

1. _____

2. _____

3. _____

CHERISH YOUR VULNERABILITY

Vulnerability can connect us, inspire us to share more deeply, and help us learn. Take a few breaths and settle into the present moment as you tune in to your body. Bring your awareness to the strong parts of your body and thank them for supporting you from one day to the next. Then, as your attention moves from one area to another, notice the *vulnerable* parts of your body. Reflect on the way vulnerability can connect you to others, inspire you to share more deeply, and help you become open to learning and transformation. Place your hands over your heart and tell your vulnerability *thank you*.

1. How does vulnerability lead to intimacy with others?

_____

_____

_____

_____

2. Do you choose to share your vulnerability with healthy people who cherish it?

_____

_____

_____

_____

3. If you are unable to share your vulnerability with others, how can you cherish it quietly within yourself?

_____

_____

_____

_____

THREE THINGS I AM GRATEFUL FOR TODAY:

1. _____

2. _____

3. _____

DAY 32

EMPOWER YOUR INTUITION WITH CONFIDENCE

To develop confidence in your intuition, cultivate an ability to connect with your felt sense of inner wisdom. With practice, you can return to your inner knowing anytime you wish, regardless of the time of day. Choose a comfortable position you can maintain for several moments. As you inhale and exhale gently with your eyes closed, tune in to your internal landscape. Imagine that with every breath, you are empowering your intuition to evolve.

1. Describe one time you listened to your intuition and you were right.

_____

_____

_____

_____

2. How does meditation strengthen your relationship with your intuition?

_____

_____

_____

_____

3. What can you do to integrate intuition more often into your daily life?

_____

_____

_____

_____

THREE THINGS I AM GRATEFUL FOR TODAY:

1. _____

2. _____

3. _____

DAY 33

PRACTICE RADICAL TRUST IN YOURSELF

Settle into a comfortable position of ease. Soften any tension. Gently inhale and exhale as you continue to breathe naturally. Imagine a space behind your mind's eye and think of one concern or negative thought that continues to trouble you this evening. Envision this concern sinking and disappearing into the vast spaciousness of your mind's eye, and let it soften into radical trust that all will be well. Give your concerns permission to dissolve, and replace them with radical self-trust.

1. Describe how it feels to trust yourself.

_____

_____

_____

_____

2. How does trusting yourself inspire others to trust you?

_____

_____

_____

_____

3. Reflect on this practice and how it feels to bring presence to the topic of self-trust.

_____

_____

_____

_____

THREE THINGS I AM GRATEFUL FOR TODAY:

1. _____

2. _____

3. _____

DAY 34

SACRED SAFETY, SACRED SLEEP

Gently close your eyes or soften your gaze and bring awareness to your breath as you settle into an easy, natural rhythm. Resting with your mouth closed, inhale and exhale effortlessly through your nose. Invite feelings of strength and sacred clarity to come to you this evening. Bring your awareness to the presence of inner strength and invite it to expand. Set an intention for your sleep to be good and centered in this gentle, quiet safety.

1. What do you notice when you tap into your inner strength?

_____

_____

_____

_____

2. How do you cultivate a sense of safety and calm for a restful evening?

_____

_____

_____

_____

3. Do you notice a shift within after completing this practice?

_____

_____

_____

_____

THREE THINGS I AM GRATEFUL FOR TODAY:

1. _____

2. _____

3. _____

DAY 35

CONNECT WITH YOUR INNER SANCTUARY

Sitting comfortably, permit an image of an inner sanctuary to form in your mind's eye. Allow the sense of this sanctuary to rest in the center of your being. Notice how beautiful it is. Let your body and the sanctuary become one. Grounded and centered in the stillness of your vast inner landscape, you are rooted in the gentle power of inner stillness. Rest here as long as you wish before continuing with your evening.

1. How does it feel to see yourself as a sanctuary?

_____

_____

_____

_____

2. Describe the qualities and sensations of your inner landscape.

_____

_____

_____

_____

3. How might you strengthen your connection to your inner sanctuary?

_____

_____

_____

_____

THREE THINGS I AM GRATEFUL FOR TODAY:

1. _____

2. _____

3. _____

DAY 36

ENVISION THE LIGHT OF POSITIVITY

Imagine luminous threads of light connecting your inner space with your outer landscape. Let nighttime sounds come and go with ease. If there are no sounds, rest in this moment of silence. As you experience the expansive connectivity between your inner and outer worlds in this moment, invite positivity to take up more space in your mind. Allow the negative emotions of the day to dissolve in this light of positivity.

1. What happens when you give yourself permission to receive joy?

_____

_____

_____

_____

2. Describe what colors and details come to mind when you visualize your light of positivity.

_____

_____

_____

_____

3. Reflect on whether you feel lighter and more prepared for restful sleep this evening.

_____

_____

_____

_____

THREE THINGS I AM GRATEFUL FOR TODAY:

1. _____

2. _____

3. _____

BEAUTY HUNTING FOR RESTORATION

The practice known as "beauty hunting," coined by author Jennifer Pastiloff, is a simple mindfulness exercise to restore inner joy. Actively searching for beauty is a transformative technique that helps you attune your mind and develop a sustainable, positive perspective. Reflect on every beautiful thing, person, or experience you encountered today. Was it a smile? A song? A loving message from a friend? Notice how it feels to be anchored in the restorative power of the beauty intrinsic to this life.

1. What beautiful things can you recall from your day?

_____

_____

_____

_____

2. How might beauty hunting as a regular practice shift your awareness?

_____

_____

_____

_____

3. Do you take time to appreciate your ability to see and sense the beauty of this life?

_____

_____

_____

_____

THREE THINGS I AM GRATEFUL FOR TODAY:

1. _____

2. _____

3. _____

DAY 38

OUT-OF-BODY MEDITATION
FOR DISSOLVING FEAR

Close your eyes and imagine rising above your body and floating gently to the ceiling. As you bring your awareness to your physical body, can you sense or see whether fear is close by? While floating above your body, invite this fear to float upward and join you in the vast space that surrounds your body with gentle stillness. Let this fear effortlessly dissolve as you float back down and return to your physical self. Embrace this state of restful ease.

1. What happens when you stop trying to push fear away and let it dissolve instead?

_____

_____

_____

_____

2. What sensations did you notice during this meditation?

_____

_____

_____

_____

3. After completing this meditation, does your body feel different or the same?

_____

_____

_____

_____

THREE THINGS I AM GRATEFUL FOR TODAY:

1. _____

2. _____

3. _____

DAY 39

INTIMACY WITH YOUR BREATH

Settle into this evening for a gentle practice of nondirective awareness, and tune in to your relationship with your breath. Without trying to become more mindful or feel more peaceful, breathe naturally as you open to the subtle quality of presence you are able to bring to each inhalation and every exhalation. As your breath emerges and dissolves without effort, imagine your breath is now breathing *you*; it is clear with gentle, abiding wisdom.

1. Are you able to find rest in the wise power of your breath?

_____

_____

_____

_____

2. Describe your relationship with your breath.

_____

_____

_____

_____

3. How can you cultivate intimacy with your breath on a regular basis?

_____

_____

_____

_____

THREE THINGS I AM GRATEFUL FOR TODAY:

1. _____

2. _____

3. _____

DAY 40

INTEND TO RECEIVE MORE OF WHAT'S GOOD FOR YOU

Start by softening your gaze and bringing awareness to your breath as you settle into an easy, natural rhythm. Resting with your mouth closed, inhale and exhale effortlessly through your nose. As you tune in to your breath this evening, connect with what is truly good in your life right now. With every inhalation and every exhalation, feel this goodness expand. Now, bring your awareness back to the present moment. Set an intention to receive more of what is good, beyond this evening and into the days ahead.

1. Reflect on and describe the things you know are good for you.

_____

_____

_____

_____

2. What actions can you take to bring more goodness into your life?

_____

_____

_____

_____

3. How do you feel about receiving more of what you deserve?

_____

_____

_____

_____

THREE THINGS I AM GRATEFUL FOR TODAY:

1. _____

2. _____

3. _____

DAY 41

GIVE YOURSELF THE REST YOU DESERVE

1. Settle into a comfortable position of ease.

2. Begin with a natural pace of inhalations and exhalations, with your mouth closed.

3. On each exhale, count slowly to six while releasing the breath through your nose.

4. On each inhale, shrug your shoulders upward toward your ears, creating a sensation of tension, then let your shoulders relax.

5. During this practice, set a clear intention to give yourself the rest you deserve.

1. What did you learn about where you store tension in your body?

_____

_____

_____

_____

2. How can you incorporate rest into your life more often?

_____

_____

_____

_____

3. What feelings and/or sensations did you notice about your breath?

_____

_____

_____

_____

THREE THINGS I AM GRATEFUL FOR TODAY:

1. _____

2. _____

3. _____

DAY 42

YOU ARE A MAGNETIC BEING
OF INFINITE POTENTIAL

Bring awareness to your breath and settle into an easy, natural rhythm.
Resting with your mouth closed, inhale and exhale effortlessly. As you tune
in to your breath this evening, connect with what you long for in your life or
how you hope to expand your potential. Perhaps it is a new job or a relationship. Whatever it may be, imagine a sense of energetic magnetism emerging
from deep within. Set a clear intention to magnetize your infinite potential
going forward.

1. What comes to mind when you pause to acknowledge your potential?

_____

_____

_____

_____

2. Does embracing your inner potential change the way you see the potential in others?

_____

_____

_____

_____

3. What quality would you like to embody more of?

_____

_____

_____

_____

THREE THINGS I AM GRATEFUL FOR TODAY:

1. _____

2. _____

3. _____

VISUALIZATION OF WORLD PEACE

Imagine a space behind your mind's eye. As this space expands, fill it with a soft, warm light. Rest in this awareness and notice an image of the world begin to emerge. Envision a healing energy surrounding the vision that rests in your mind's eye. As you begin to emanate and reflect a luminosity that is reflected back to you from golden threads that connect you with your vision of the entire world, imagine another thread of light connecting every living creature and linking all of existence in a healing, pulsing energy that carries on through the night.

1. What did you see in your visualization of world peace?

_____

_____

_____

_____

2. Based on your inspiration from this meditation, what is one action step you can take toward finding peace?

_____

_____

_____

_____

3. How does it feel to hold a vision for world peace within your
physical body?

_____

_____

_____

_____

THREE THINGS I AM GRATEFUL FOR TODAY:

1. _____

2. _____

3. _____

DAY 44

RELEASE WHAT YOU DID NOT FINISH TODAY

Bring your attention to the day behind you, and mentally travel back in time. In your mind's eye, notice what you did not complete. Did you learn that you needed more time than you actually gave yourself for appointments, responsibilities, or travel in between meetings? Set an intention to release self-judgment and begin anew tomorrow. Make a conscious choice to tune in to ways you can alter your schedule and manage time with fluid ease.

1. How does it feel to let go of what you did not complete today?

_____

_____

_____

_____

2. As you become more present, what do you notice about your ability to manage time with wisdom?

_____

_____

_____

_____

3. Does understanding you can begin again tomorrow help you prepare for a restful evening?

_____

_____

_____

_____

THREE THINGS I AM GRATEFUL FOR TODAY:

1. _____

2. _____

3. _____

DAY 45

THE WISDOM OF RENEWAL

Choose a comfortable position you can maintain for several moments. Bring your attention to tomorrow, then mentally travel into your future. If any thoughts or feelings of anxiety about the day ahead arise, simply allow them to pass from your awareness on their own, maintaining a gentle rhythm of your breath. In your mind's eye, reflect on your stamina and take time to contemplate your schedule. How often do you rest? Make a conscious choice to recharge more often; sleep, rest, and quietude are essential to the body's instinct to renew itself.

4. What sensations did you notice during this practice?

_____

_____

_____

_____

5. How strong is your faith in your body's capacity to renew itself?

_____

_____

_____

_____

6. Reflect on what might happen if you harness your body's wisdom of renewal.

_____

_____

_____

_____

THREE THINGS I AM GRATEFUL FOR TODAY:

1. _____

2. _____

3. _____

DAY 46

SOCIAL MEDIA FAST FOR EVENING PEACE

Smartphones and other technology devices are known to cause anxiety, stress, and varying degrees of emotional unease. Take time to reflect on the media you consume in the evening. For a few moments, tune in to your body and settle into the ease and quality of your breath. Call to your mind how it might feel to replace this consumption with more rest. Set an intention to limit your media intake by turning off all tech two hours before you plan to go to sleep. Give yourself the gift of stillness.

1. What physical sensations do you notice when you disconnect from technology?

_____

_____

_____

_____

2. How can you protect yourself from the stress and anxiety of social media?

_____

_____

_____

_____

3. Do you find it difficult to give yourself time away from electronics before you prepare for sleep?

_____

_____

_____

_____

THREE THINGS I AM GRATEFUL FOR TODAY:

1. _____
2. _____
3. _____

DAY 47

MINDFUL BREATHING FOR SELF-HEALING

1. When thoughts or feelings seem overwhelming, mindful breathing is a support. Rest in a comfortable space and bring your attention to your breath.

2. As you inhale and exhale naturally, invite your breath to be fluid and come and go with ease.

3. Allow negative thoughts and feelings of judgment to rest inside your breath and be expelled with each exhalation.

4. Experience the stillness and feelings of peace that come with mindful breathing.

1. Describe your relationship with your breath when you apply the wisdom of your breath to self-healing.

_____

_____

_____

_____

2. How does it feel to invoke your capacity to practice self-healing?

_____

_____

_____

_____

3. What happens when you pause self-judgment and let feelings or thoughts rest inside your breath?

_____

_____

_____

_____

THREE THINGS I AM GRATEFUL FOR TODAY:

1. _____

2. _____

3. _____

YOUR BODY POWERS UP WHILE YOU SLEEP

Find a comfortable, quiet place. Resting your hands wherever you wish, relax your fingers and loosen your jaw. As you soften your gaze or close your eyes, tap into the rhythm of your breath and bring to your mind's eye a quiet, powerful warmth nestling deep within the center of your body. Visualize this warmth expanding. Let your body relax, one breath at a time, and notice the strong, good presence of self-love. Restore your connection and invite your sleep to fully recharge you.

1. How might you change your lifestyle to incorporate more sleep going forward?

_____

_____

_____

_____

2. If you could gain one superpower while you sleep, what would it be and why?

_____

_____

_____

_____

3. How does it feel to trust your body's ability to restore itself?

_____

_____

_____

_____

THREE THINGS I AM GRATEFUL FOR TODAY:

1. _____

2. _____

3. _____

DAY 49

MEDITATION FOR SOFTENING NEGATIVE EMOTIONS

Rest quietly and connect with the present moment. Anchor into the center of your being as you reflect on the powerful sensations of negative emotions in your body that may linger from your day. Explore these emotions without self-judgment and tune in to the energy behind them. As an experiment, ask yourself if these emotions can be softened. Let the sensations of these emotions rest beside you without pushing them away. Practice the art of mindful attention and meet yourself with presence this evening.

1. What happens when you invite negative emotions to soften instead of pushing them away?

_____

_____

_____

_____

2. If your anger could speak, what would it tell you it needs?

_____

_____

_____

_____

3. How does it feel to explore your negative emotions without judgment?

_____

_____

_____

_____

THREE THINGS I AM GRATEFUL FOR TODAY:

1. _____

2. _____

3. _____

DAY 50

FIND PURPOSE IN SHARING LOVE WITH OTHERS

Perhaps you were conditioned to believe you are unworthy of love or cannot be loved because of unresolved wounds. In truth, our neurological systems are hardwired to thrive, transform, and evolve in the safety of healthy relationships; as feeling creatures that think, there is purpose to be discovered in sharing our love with others we care for, cherish, and trust. Take time to attune to the present moment this evening and cast off the belief you must be more or less; we belong to each other.

1. How much time do you dedicate to building healthy relationships?

_____

_____

_____

_____

2. What changes can you make to your lifestyle to spend less time in isolation?

_____

_____

_____

_____

3. What action can you take to make more space for love in your life?

_____

_____

_____

_____

THREE THINGS I AM GRATEFUL FOR TODAY:

1. _____

2. _____

3. _____

DAY 51

ENERGY OF PEACE

Close your eyes and imagine a soft white light floating before you. As it gets near enough for you to touch its outer perimeter, permit yourself to slip inside it. As you move into this energy of healing and peace, take note of any emotions or sensations that may arise. What feelings are you made aware of? Remain in this energy for as long as you wish to this evening. Explore your invisible layer of peace.

1. Reflect on your experience of this meditation.

_____

_____

_____

_____

2. Describe the sensations you experienced within your energy of peace.

_____

_____

_____

_____

3. How might you be able to cultivate this energy of peace in your day tomorrow?

_____

_____

_____

_____

THREE THINGS I AM GRATEFUL FOR TODAY:

1. _____

2. _____

3. _____

CHOOSE TO RECEIVE MORE JOY

Imagine a warm sensation of joy expanding from your heart this evening, and center yourself in your breath. With every inhalation and every exhalation, imagine yourself connecting with the loved ones in your life as you tune in to an experience of spontaneous joy without cause. Continue to be enveloped by a current of empathetic connectivity as you let yourself breathe naturally. Starting tomorrow, open yourself up to supporting or receiving support from others as needed.

1. How does it feel to make a conscious choice to open yourself to joy?

_____

_____

_____

_____

2. What does joy feel like to you, emotionally and physically?

_____

_____

_____

_____

3. What changes can you make in your life to receive more joy?

_____

_____

_____

_____

THREE THINGS I AM GRATEFUL FOR TODAY:

1. _____

2. _____

3. _____

DAY 53

TURN WORRY INTO WISDOM

Rest quietly and connect with the present moment. Anchor into the center of your being. Notice any sensation of worry that feels overwhelming or intrusive this evening. Where is the tension of worry living in your body, right now? Explore this physical experience without self-judgment. As an experiment, ask yourself if this worry can be transformed into somatic wisdom. In other words, what good action might you take tomorrow? What is worry revealing about your inner wisdom?

1. What do you notice about the relationship between worry and wisdom?

_____

_____

_____

_____

2. How can feeling worried inspire you to take wise action?

_____

_____

_____

_____

3. If your worry could speak, what would it say it needs from you?

_____

_____

_____

_____

THREE THINGS I AM GRATEFUL FOR TODAY:

1. _____

2. _____

3. _____

DAY 54

CELEBRATE YOUR RESILIENCE

With your eyes either open or closed, ground yourself in the present moment. Bring to mind a difficult or overwhelming emotion you experienced during your day. Inhale and exhale through your nose in an easy, natural rhythm with your mouth closed. While gently holding this emotion in your mind's eye, allow your inner resilience to fully envelop the difficult emotion you just recalled, and observe as the emotion slowly dissolves. Celebrate your resilience and the support it brings you.

1. How often do you take time to celebrate how far you've come?

_____

_____

_____

_____

2. When you celebrate your resilience, how does that change the way you see resilience in others?

_____

_____

_____

_____

3. How can you choose to strengthen your resilience?

_____

_____

_____

_____

THREE THINGS I AM GRATEFUL FOR TODAY:

1. _____

2. _____

3. _____

DAY 55

RECONNECT WITH YOUR SOUL

Begin tonight's meditation by imagining a space behind your mind's eye. As it expands, permit yourself to receive the gift of spontaneous inspiration this evening and in the days ahead. Rest in the awareness that instinctual creativity is grounded in gentle presence; you can tap into it anytime. Notice if any particular thoughts or ideas come to mind. As often as possible, reconnect with your soul and be mindful of its needs.

1. What special characteristics do you notice about your soul?

_____

_____

_____

_____

2. How does your soul protect and empower you, even when you are unaware?

_____

_____

_____

_____

3. If your soul could give you a message right now, what would
that message be?

_____

_____

_____

_____

THREE THINGS I AM GRATEFUL FOR TODAY:

1. _____

2. _____

3. _____

DAY 56

ABIDING WITH WHAT IS

To abide means to accept. The contemplative practice of abiding is a no-nonsense approach to meditation that consists, quite literally, of sitting with what is, without trying to change anything. For the next several moments, rest in natural awareness of the present moment. Allow your thoughts or emotions of the day behind you to come to mind this evening. If you find you feel physically uncomfortable, shift your position until you feel at ease. Abiding with what is can be surprisingly transformative.

1. Reflect on how an abiding practice can help you rest in the moment.

_____

_____

_____

_____

2. How does mindful breathing act as a support for an abiding practice?

_____

_____

_____

_____

3. How does taking small breaks from trying to change the world help you recharge?

_____

_____

_____

_____

THREE THINGS I AM GRATEFUL FOR TODAY:

1. _____

2. _____

3. _____

THE INTELLIGENCE OF YOUR HEARTBEAT

This meditation is done lying down with eyes closed. Gently scan your body for sensations, beginning with your fingers and toes. As you inhale and exhale, move your attention toward your heart. As you rest your awareness in the center of the innermost chambers of your heart, continue to breathe mindfully for several moments and tune in to your heartbeat. With every inhalation, feel the pulse of intelligence in your heart. With every exhalation, allow feelings of negativity about your day to dissolve. Carry this rhythm into sleep and rest with ease.

1. Reflect on your experience with this meditation.

_____

_____

_____

_____

2. What did you discover about the intelligence of your heart?

_____

_____

_____

_____

3. What might happen if your heart intelligence and your intellectual intelligence are in sync?

_____

_____

_____

_____

THREE THINGS I AM GRATEFUL FOR TODAY:

1. _____

2. _____

3. _____

TONGLEN TO TRANSFORM SUFFERING

The Tibetan practice of *tonglen* is the act of changing suffering into compassion by working consciously with the intelligence of your breath. With every inhale (*len*, accepting), imagine inhaling the energy of suffering. With every exhale (*Tong*, sending out), imagine this suffering has been transformed by your breath; that same energy is now an outpouring of warm, compassionate presence. *Tonglen* is a way to metabolize the energy of suffering, then turn it into compassion.

1. How does it feel to recognize your breath as a transformative resource?

_____

_____

_____

_____

2. What comes to mind when you hear the phrase "be the change you wish to see"?

_____

_____

_____

_____

3. What do you notice in your body after practicing *tonglen*?

_____

_____

_____

_____

THREE THINGS I AM GRATEFUL FOR TODAY:

1. _____

2. _____

3. _____

DAY 59

BOX BREATHING FOR STRESS RELIEF

Also known as square breathing, this meditation practice helps you calm the nervous system, improve concentration, and/or prepare for rest. There are four distinct parts:

1. Exhale through your nose with your mouth closed (to gently expel all air from your inner landscape).

2. Slowly inhale to a count of four.

3. While holding this breath, count to four again.

4. Slowly exhale this breath while counting to four. Repeat as often as you wish.

1. What impact does this practice have on your level of stress or anxiety?

_____

_____

_____

_____

2. Did the quality of your breathing change in any noticeable way?

_____

_____

_____

_____

3. How can you use this practice at different times to help manage stress?

_____

_____

_____

_____

THREE THINGS I AM GRATEFUL FOR TODAY:

1. _____

2. _____

3. _____

CHERISH YOUR ABILITY TO TRANSFORM

As human beings, we tend to forget our ability to transform is extraordinary—and meant to be cherished. Without controlling your breath, gently inhale and exhale. Close your eyes and notice a sensation of calm that rests in the space *between* your thoughts. Tune in to this space in your mind's eye and take this time to bring a sense of caring presence to your evening. Offer a quiet, simple prayer of gratitude for your ability to attune to your inner wisdom and transform as often as necessary.

1. When you realize the very nature of your being is transformative, how does this change the way you see yourself?

_____

_____

_____

_____

2. How does it feel to work intimately and proactively with your neuroplasticity?

_____

_____

_____

_____

3. If consciousness is creative, what does this mean for your ability to shift your awareness as needed?

_____

_____

_____

_____

THREE THINGS I AM GRATEFUL FOR TODAY:

1. _____

2. _____

3. _____

DAY 61

MIRRORLIKE WISDOM

The true nature of your mind rests in mirrorlike wisdom. This does *not* mean every thought or feeling is an obscuration. What it does mean is this: Each night before you close your day, it is a good practice to envision yourself clearing the mirror of your mind's eye so you awaken truly refreshed. While resting in a comfortable position, imagine your mind as a mirror. With every breath, envision this mirror becoming more clear, more polished.

1. What comes to mind when you think of mirrorlike wisdom?

_____

_____

_____

_____

2. How does it feel to "polish" your thoughts, feelings, and innermost perspective?

_____

_____

_____

_____

3. What happens when you see your mind as your ally and not your enemy?

_____

_____

_____

_____

THREE THINGS I AM GRATEFUL FOR TODAY:

1. _____

2. _____

3. _____

ECSTATIC DANCE FOR RELEASING ANXIETY

Ecstatic dance can revitalize the brain's ability to process creativity; joy associated with this type of practice has been shown to activate the dopamine/opioid reward system. So if you're feeling anxious, it might be a good time to shake it all out! Choose upbeat music you love and dance for several songs, as if nobody is watching. As you wind down for the evening, imagine that with every move you make, you are releasing anxiety and restoring inner flow.

1. What physical sensations do you notice after shaking anxiety loose?

_____

_____

_____

_____

2. Now that your anxiety has been released into the atmosphere, what can you focus on instead?

_____

_____

_____

_____

3. How does it feel to make meditation more fun instead of being more serious?

_____

_____

_____

_____

THREE THINGS I AM GRATEFUL FOR TODAY:

1. _____

2. _____

3. _____

DAY 63

PRAYER OF THE EMPTY BOWL

At the end of the day, we can feel empty and drained. This meditation practice is a visualization; it is a contemplative moment in which you fully acknowledge a feeling of "having nothing left." Close your eyes and assume a natural rhythm with your breath. Imagine an empty bowl, and then visualize this emptiness being filled by healing energy. Whenever you feel empty, envision a healing light pouring into you from the crown of your head. Imagine that every cell of your being is filled with new boundless strength.

1. During this visualization, what did you imagine your healing energy looks like?

_____

_____

_____

_____

2. In times of great distress, how do you take time to replenish your inner resources?

_____

_____

_____

_____

3. In moments of extreme exhaustion, how do you feel about trusting a divine strength you can tap in to anytime?

_____

_____

_____

_____

THREE THINGS I AM GRATEFUL FOR TODAY:

1. _____

2. _____

3. _____

DAY 64

CULTIVATE APPRECIATION

Voicing appreciation aloud is a mindful way to close a day and attune to your language of love while preparing for rest and sleep. Set aside time for reflecting on what you appreciate most about a family member, loved one, or friend. At the same time, reflect on how you think that person would voice their appreciation about you. Try to be specific and as honest as possible.

1. How does it feel to cultivate appreciation?

_____

_____

_____

_____

2. What feels good about being seen and appreciated by someone else?

_____

_____

_____

_____

3. How does it feel to actively offer appreciation to someone you care about?

_____

_____

_____

_____

THREE THINGS I AM GRATEFUL FOR TODAY:

1. _____

2. _____

3. _____

SIMPLE MANTRA FOR OVERALL WELL-BEING

Research shows a simple mantra practice can improve your overall sense of well-being. Settle into a comfortable position and silently repeat the following with eyes open or closed. Try doing this for several minutes. Allow thoughts reflecting on the trials of the day to come and go.

I am a good person. I deserve to feel healthy, happy, and whole.
I am a good person. I deserve to feel healthy, happy, and whole.
I am a good person. I deserve to feel healthy, happy, and whole.

1. Take time to reflect on how you feel after completing this practice.

_____

_____

_____

_____

2. Which part of the mantra do you feel you need to hear more of?

_____

_____

_____

_____

3. In times of stress, how can a mantra practice like this help you feel stronger?

_____

_____

_____

_____

THREE THINGS I AM GRATEFUL FOR TODAY:

1. _____

2. _____

3. _____

DAY 66

SAY GOODBYE TO THIS DAY

A resistance to the changeable nature of this life or the impermanence of time can lead to feelings of anguish and sorrow. This is completely normal (and marvelously human). Experiment with grounding yourself in impermanence by consciously saying goodbye to this day. Reflect with appreciation on what you loved most or how you passed your time. By acknowledging that today will never return, you learn to face impermanence with compassion and real courage.

1. How does it feel to face impermanence with courage?

_____

_____

_____

_____

2. When you acknowledge the passing of time, how does that change the way you live?

_____

_____

_____

_____

3. Do you think that grieving a little bit each day might help you be more open to the joy of this life?

_____

_____

_____

_____

THREE THINGS I AM GRATEFUL FOR TODAY:

1. _____

2. _____

3. _____

EMBRACE THIS BEAUTIFUL MESS

Many of us are conditioned to believe we should focus on specific emotions such as love, joy, positivity, and other feelings commonly associated with spiritually "advanced" states of awareness. In truth, a devotion to *feeling everything* is the true path of the heart. When we make peace with this life as a beautiful, shattering mess, there is no right or wrong way to live. With every breath, embrace your beautiful mess with presence.

1. How does it feel to fully relinquish the idea of perfection when it comes to living?

_____

_____

_____

_____

2. If you see the mess as beautiful, does this allow you to become more aware of possibilities? Why or why not?

_____

_____

_____

_____

3. What happens when you decide to hug your mess?

_____

_____

_____

_____

THREE THINGS I AM GRATEFUL FOR TODAY:

1. _____

2. _____

3. _____

DAY 68

INTEND TO STOP HATING YOUR MIND

Silencing or rejecting your cognitive, thinking intelligence is a self-destructive habit; neuroplasticity is a miraculous, elegant resource that can be harnessed—if you choose to *stop hating your mind*. Challenge yourself to practice STOP if you find yourself judging thoughts. Allow these thoughts to fade away with each exhalation.

1. *Silence* the inner critic.

2. *Tell* your mind you *love* its capacity to transform.

3. *Open* yourself to seeing yourself as *highly* intelligent.

4. *Practice* mindful breathing to restore calm self-love.

1. How can this practice help you harness the power of your mind?

_____

_____

_____

_____

2. If you knew your mind was your most powerful ally, how would that change the way you see yourself?

_____

_____

_____

_____

3. If you knew that neuroplasticity was your most important resource, would you prioritize meditation as an act of self-care?

_____

_____

_____

_____

THREE THINGS I AM GRATEFUL FOR TODAY:

1. _____

2. _____

3. _____

DAY 69

COHERENT BREATHING PRACTICE FOR LOSS

Have you—or someone you know—experienced unexpected loss? Perhaps you are grieving. Sometimes the best practice is the simple one. Tonight, give yourself the grace to be exactly where you are. Tune out the world for a few minutes as you practice coherent breathing with your mouth closed: Inhale while counting slowly to six, then exhale while counting slowly to six. Let the spacious intelligence of your breath hold you in abiding, kindhearted warmth.

1. What happens when you let your breath hold your grief?

_____

_____

_____

_____

2. How often do you take time to rest in times of loss or anguish?

_____

_____

_____

_____

3. If your grief could speak, what would it say it needs?

_____

_____

_____

_____

THREE THINGS I AM GRATEFUL FOR TODAY:

1. _____

2. _____

3. _____

DAY 70

REVIEW THE PAST, THEN LOOK TOWARD THE FUTURE

The spectacular ability of your thinking, conscious mind to solve problems, overcome obstacles, and dream bigger is its nature. We review past experiences in order to look toward the future with greater awareness. Take time to reflect on what you discovered today about what worked and what didn't, without judgment. Now, envision in your mind's eye what you hope to do differently tomorrow. The past can be informative; look toward the future with vision.

1. Reflect on your experience of today and what you learned.

_____

_____

_____

_____

2. What wisdom from today can you take with you into the future?

_____

_____

_____

_____

3. What feelings of self-judgment can you release and leave behind?

_____

_____

_____

_____

THREE THINGS I AM GRATEFUL FOR TODAY:

1. _____

2. _____

3. _____

DOODLING/COLORING MEDITATION FOR CREATIVE FLOW

Doodling or coloring can help us wind down in the evening with creative flow. If you have a coloring book, grab some art materials, turn on your favorite music, and ease into this autotelic meditation. If you don't have a coloring book, doodle! Grab any piece of paper you can find and set a timer for 60 seconds. Without thinking, start doodling. Don't let your pen or pencil leave the paper for the entire minute, then see what emerges.

1. How does it feel to do a creative and mindless activity to become more mindful?

_____

_____

_____

_____

2. Was this practice fun? Why or why not?

_____

_____

_____

_____

3. If you doodled, what shapes did you create? Was there any meaning behind them?

_____

_____

_____

_____

THREE THINGS I AM GRATEFUL FOR TODAY:

1. _____

2. _____

3. _____

DAY 72

METTA FOR LIVING WITH CHRONIC ILLNESS OR PAIN

Metta is loosely translated as "loving, kind, or generous with goodwill." If you live with chronic illness or pain, or take care of someone who does, this practice can be deeply restorative. At the end of your day, take time to notice feelings of compassion fatigue, exhaustion, or frustration. While breathing gently, repeat the following: *May I be kind to myself. May I be kind to others. May I be at ease.* With each exhale, let sensations of discomfort dissolve.

1. How does cherishing yourself with loving-kindness feel?

_____

_____

_____

_____

2. How did this practice help you dissolve feelings of frustration, anger, or anxiety?

_____

_____

_____

_____

3. How does it feel to know you can practice this anytime, anywhere, for any reason to offer yourself the patient love you truly deserve?

_____

_____

_____

_____

THREE THINGS I AM GRATEFUL FOR TODAY:

1. _____

2. _____

3. _____

DAY 73

CELEBRATE YOUR NEEDS

Because we are interdependent beings who need each other, the practice of asking for what we need is a powerful, celebratory practice. Recall the events of today, soften your gaze, and bring awareness to your breath while centering yourself within. Inhale and exhale gently as you connect with your ability to ask for what you need. If this is a skill you need to practice, set an intention to do so with someone you trust.

1. What happens when you celebrate your needs instead of sacrificing them?

_____

_____

_____

_____

2. Does the practice of celebrating your needs change the way you see the needs of others?

_____

_____

_____

_____

3. What is one tangible way you would like to celebrate one of your needs?

_____

_____

_____

_____

THREE THINGS I AM GRATEFUL FOR TODAY:

1. _____
2. _____
3. _____

DAY 74

VISUALIZATION FOR DISSOLVING PHYSICAL PAIN

As you soften your gaze or close your eyes, visualize a part of your body where you feel physical pain this evening. Tune in to your breath and imagine that you are weightless, as if you are floating in space. With each breath, notice this space expanding and invite your physical pain to float with you, as if it, too, is weightless, afloat. In the heart of this spacious awareness, connect with the vastness within, and breathe with gentle ease.

1. What happens when you take time to let physical pain dissolve?

_____

_____

_____

_____

2. If your physical pain did not change, how can you hold yourself in radical self-love?

_____

_____

_____

_____

3. How would you describe your relationship with pain, and how can you nurture yourself more?

_____

_____

_____

_____

THREE THINGS I AM GRATEFUL FOR TODAY:

1. _____

2. _____

3. _____

DAY 75

SETTING INTENTIONS FOR TOMORROW

Setting an intention for tomorrow supports the brain's natural instinct to focus on something tangible. Take time to think through the day you've already had, then imagine the day ahead. As you lean into your vision for tomorrow, set a clear intention for how you hope to feel. Then, set a clear intention for at least one action step you will take first thing in the morning to nourish the feeling you want to experience.

1. How do you hope to feel tomorrow?

_____

_____

_____

_____

2. What action will you take to support that feeling?

_____

_____

_____

_____

3. How does it feel to look ahead and plan for what you want to experience?

_____

_____

_____

_____

THREE THINGS I AM GRATEFUL FOR TODAY:

1. _____

2. _____

3. _____

DAY 76

RELEASE TENSION WITH PROGRESSIVE MUSCLE RELAXATION

Lying down in a comfortable position, let gravity hold you in weighted, calm awareness. Beginning with your toes, clench your muscles so they tense up, then release. Then, do the same with your ankles and fingers. Clench your jaw, your facial muscles, and your mouth, then release them and let them relax. Move gradually from the outer edges of your body and repeat this practice until you reach your core muscles. Rest quietly for several moments, allowing thoughts of the day and self-judgment to dissolve.

1. Reflect on this practice.

_____

_____

_____

_____

2. Where do you store the most tension, and why do you think that is?

_____

_____

_____

_____

3. Which part of you feels the most relaxed? How can you support your need for relaxation in the future?

_____

_____

_____

_____

THREE THINGS I AM GRATEFUL FOR TODAY:

1. _____

2. _____

3. _____

DAY 77

BRINGING WARMTH TO SENSATIONS OF LONELINESS

While breathing naturally, imagine a feeling of calm, peace, or simple warmth beginning to fill every space in your body. Beginning with the top of your head, imagine it moving through your entire being until you feel a sense of warmth, peace, and heartfelt presence. Feel an even greater warmth expanding in the center of your being and sense it permeating your loneliness, as if there is a tiny, radiant star shining from within.

1. What do you notice as you bring warmth to the sensation of loneliness?

_____

_____

_____

_____

2. What action steps can you take to build more connection into your life?

_____

_____

_____

_____

3. How does it feel knowing that you can self-generate warmth when you need it most?

_____

_____

_____

_____

THREE THINGS I AM GRATEFUL FOR TODAY:

1. _____

2. _____

3. _____

DAY 78

HEARTMIND® MEDITATION FOR ANXIETY

Resting your hands where they are most comfortable, settle into a relaxed position, and invite grace into this moment, into your body. Notice the flow of your breath soften naturally and move with ease. Gathering your awareness to your heart, mind, and breath, bring your awareness to the integrated presence of your innermost HeartMind® intelligence. Then, locate the feeling of anxiety in your body. With every exhale, release this anxiety. Attune yourself to sensations of calm.

1. When you tune in to your heart, mind, and breath, are you able to notice the quiet, calming power of your inner landscape?

_____

_____

_____

_____

2. What happens to your experience of anxiety when you attend to it with kindness?

_____

_____

_____

_____

3. How often do you tell yourself how proud you are of yourself for managing stress and challenges?

_____

_____

_____

_____

THREE THINGS I AM GRATEFUL FOR TODAY:

1. _____

2. _____

3. _____

DAY 79

DREAM BIGGER TO BUILD COURAGE

Many of us are afraid to dream, because dreaming takes courage. However, dreaming also *builds* courage. Invite yourself to consider this possibility: If your greatest dream is bigger than your deepest fear, perhaps moving forward will be less frightening—and more exciting. With each breath, take a moment to integrate a deep sense of belonging and intimacy with yourself. Tune in to your most important dream. Give yourself permission to have real faith in your potential.

1. What dream do you have that is bigger than your fear?

_____

_____

_____

_____

2. What small steps can you take to make this dream come true?

_____

_____

_____

_____

3. If you knew confidence was built by taking action, do you think you would take action more often?

_____

_____

_____

_____

THREE THINGS I AM GRATEFUL FOR TODAY:

1. _____

2. _____

3. _____

"WHEREVER YOU ARE IS THE ENTRY POINT."

—*Kabir*

PARTING WORDS

By returning to the sanctuary that rests within, you have traveled the path of spiritual homecoming. This requires courage, skill, and remarkable faith—in *yourself*. Take a moment to celebrate this experience and embrace physical wellness and your newfound awareness. By taking a meditation journey such as the one you just completed, you built new neural networks, engaged a gratitude practice to enhance your well-being, and, in a very short time, reconnected with the most powerful technology in the world: your inner landscape. As I often say to my clients and meditation students, when you begin to nourish your meditation practice, your meditation practice begins to nourish you.

The specific meditation practice does not matter. How long you practice does not matter. What *does* matter is whether you consciously devote several minutes, every day, to connecting with the sophisticated nature of your being, because this inner technology is meant to be activated whenever necessary for recovery, renewal, and restoration. Since you now see that your entire being functions at the elegant nexus of somatic intelligence and soulful presence, the most transformative work you can do is *harness the powerful resource that is you*. In essence, as you become the change you seek and embody natural, awakened presence, you touch others with a felt sense of your humanity, without even trying. When we discover the lantern within, we recognize the light that exists in others, and by meeting the sacred territory of unbound potential, our path of luminosity is spontaneously realized, one breath at a time. To illuminate this life with mindful awareness, to rest deeply and live wakefully from the heart of your remembrance, is a gift to the world.

RESOURCES

BOOKS

Brown, Richard P., and Patricia L. Gerbarg. *The Healing Power of the Breath: Simple Techniques to Reduce Stress and Anxiety, Enhance Concentration, and Balance Your Emotions.* Boston: Shambhala, 2012.

Clear, James. *Atomic Habits: An Easy & Proven Way to Build Good Habits & Break Bad Ones.* New York: Avery, 2018.

Gillihan, Seth J. *The CBT Deck: 101 Practices to Improve Thoughts, Be in the Moment & Take Action in Your Life.* Eau Claire: PESI, 2019.

Harris, Dan. *10% Happier: How I Tamed the Voice in My Head, Reduced Stress without Losing My Edge, and Found Self-Help That Actually Works—A True Story.* New York: Dey Street, 2014.

Rinpoche, Tenzin Wangyal. *Tibetan Sound Healing: Seven Guided Practices for Clearing Obstacles, Accessing Positive Qualities, and Uncovering Your Inherent Wisdom.* N.p.: Sounds True, 2020.

Siegel, Daniel J. *Aware: The Science and Practice of Presence.* New York: TarcherPerigee, 2018.

ONLINE

Insight Timer (InsightTimer.com)
App and online community for meditation.

Headspace (Headspace.com)
App for mindfulness and meditation.

Tara Brach (TaraBrach.com)
Website of psychologist and meditation teacher Tara Brach, with several meditations and other resources.

Recovery Dharma (RecoveryDharma.org)
Buddhist-based program and fellowship for recovery from addiction.

REFERENCES

Bailey, Jenny. "Beauty Hunting: Finding the Magic in Your Every Day Life." Medium, December 4, 2019. medium.com/@jennybailey14/beauty-hunting-finding-the-magic-in-your-every-day-life-fc9f5143e3f1/.

Black, David S., and George M. Slavich. "Mindfulness Meditation and the Immune System: A Systematic Review of Randomized Controlled Trials." *Annals of the New York Academy of Sciences* 1373, no. 1 (June 2016): 13–24. doi.org/10.1111/nyas.12998.

Brach, Tara. "Feeling Overwhelmed? Remember RAIN." Mindful, February 7, 2019. mindful.org/tara-brach-rain-mindfulness-practice/.

Chödrön, Pema. *Tonglen: The Path of Transformation*. N.p.: Vajradhatu Publications, 2001.

Hagerty, Michael R., Julian Isaacs, Leigh Brasington, Larry Shupe, Eberhard E. Fetz, and Steven C. Cramer. "Case Study of Ecstatic Meditation: fMRI and EEG Evidence of Self-Stimulating a Reward System." *Neural Plasticity* 2013 (May 2013): 1–12. doi.org/10.1155/2013/653572.

Lolla, Aruna. "Mantras Help the General Psychological Well-Being of College Students: A Pilot Study." *Journal of Religion and Health* 57 (March 2017): 110–119. doi.org/10.1007/s10943-017-0371-7.

Ong, Jason C., and Christine E. Smith. "Using Mindfulness for the Treatment of Insomnia." *Current Sleep Medicine Reports* 3 (April 2017): 57–65. doi.org/10.1007/s40675-017-0068-1.

Rinpoche, Tenzin Wangyal. "Tenzin Wangyal on the Five Indestructible Warrior Sounds." Shambhala Publications. Accessed January 2021. shambhala.com/snowlion_articles/the-five-indestructible-warrior-sounds/.

Stokes, Worthy. Insight Timer. Accessed January 2021. InsightTimer.com/WorthyStokes.

ABOUT THE AUTHOR

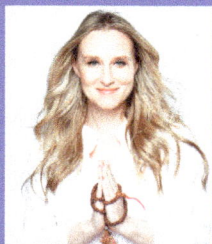

WORTHY STOKES is a bestselling author and the founder of The HeartMind® Process. Her warm, personable teaching style reflects an embodied spiritual perspective that is grounded in years of advanced contemplative practice, and her guided HeartMind® meditations have touched thousands across the world. Learn more about her at WorthyStokes.com.